COMPLETE GUIDE TO UNDERSTANDING COCHLEAR IMPLANT SURGERY

Mastering Scala Media, A Detailed Handbook On Procedures, Techniques, And Postoperative Care For Enhanced Hearing Restoration

KLEIN HOYLE

© [KLEIN HOYLE] [2024]

All rights reserved.

No part of this book may be reproduced, distributed, or transmitted in any form or by any means, including photocopying, recording, or other electronic or mechanical methods, without the publisher's prior written permission, with the exception of brief quotations in critical reviews and certain other noncommercial uses permitted by copyright law.

Disclaimer

The content in this book is based on the author's expertise and comprehension of the topic. The author has no affiliation or link with any corporation, business, or person. This book is meant to give general information and educational material only, and it should not be interpreted as professional medical advice. Always seek the advice of a skilled healthcare expert if you have any queries about medical issues or treatments. The author and publisher expressly disclaim any responsibility resulting directly or indirectly from the use or use of the information included in this book.

Table of Contents

CHAPTER 1 15
- Introduction To Cochlear Implant Surgery 15
- What Is A Cochlear Implant? 15
- How Do Cochlear Implants Work? 15
- Who Is Suitable For Cochlear Implant Surgery? . 17
- Overview Of The Surgical Procedure 18

CHAPTER 2 21
- Preparing For Cochlear Implant Surgery 21
- The Consultation And Evaluation Process 21
- Medical Tests And Assessments 22
  - 1. Imaging Studies: 23
  - 3. Balance Testing: 23
  - 4. Psychological examination: 24
- Preoperative Instructions and Guidelines 24
  - 1. Medication Guidelines: 24
  - 2. Fasting Instructions: 25
  - 3. Hygiene Protocol: 25
  - 4. Arrangements for Transportation and Accompaniment: 25
- Mental And Emotional Preparation 26

1. Educate Them: 26
2. Seek Support: 26
3. Practice Relaxation Techniques: 27
4. Communicate with Healthcare professionals: 27

CHAPTER 3 29
Surgical Procedure 29
Anesthesia And Incision 29
Installation Of The Implant Device 30
Secure The Electrode Array 31
Closing The Incision And Postoperative Care ...32

CHAPTER 4 35
Recovery And Rehabilitation 35
Immediate Post-Op Care............................35
Healing Process And Follow-Up Appointments .36
Activation Of The Cochlear Implant 37
Auditory Training And Rehabilitation Programs 38

CHAPTER 5 41
Potential Risks And Complications 41
Surgery Risks And Precautions 41
Device-Related Complications 42

Strategies For Minimizing Risk 43

Long-Term Monitoring And Management 44

CHAPTER 6 47

Adjusting To Life With A Cochlear Implant 47

Expectations Vs Reality 47

Adapting To Sound Perception 48

Communication Strategies And Speech Therapy 49

Lifestyle Changes And Support Networks 50

CHAPTER 7 53

Maintenance And Care For The Cochlear Implant
.... 53

Daily Care Routine For External Components ... 53

2. Battery Management: 54

4. Securing the Processor: 54

5. Check for Damage: 54

Troubleshooting: Common Issues 55

3. Discomfort or Irritation: 56

4. Loss of Connection: 56

5. Inconsistent Performance: 57

Battery Management And Replacement 57

1. Rechargeable Batteries: 57

2. Disposable Batteries: 58

3. Battery Life: 58

4. Emergency Preparedness: 58

5. Battery Replacement: 59

Regular Device Checks And Maintenance 59

1. Monitoring Performance: 60

2. Troubleshooting Issues: 60

3. Device Maintenance: 60

4. Counseling and assistance: 61

5. Long-term Monitoring: 61

CHAPTER 8 63

Maximizing The Benefits Of Cochlear Implants . 63

Continued Auditory Training And Rehabilitation
....63

Exploring Advanced Features And Accessories .. 64

Strategies For Challenged Listening Environments
....65

Advocacy And Community Involvement 67

CHAPTER 9 69

Financial Considerations And Insurance Coverage
....69

Cost Of Cochlear Implant Surgery 69
Insurance Coverage And Reimbursement 70
Financial Assistance Programs 71
Planning For Long-Term Maintenance Expenses 71
CHAPTER 10 73
Future Developments And Emerging Technology 73
Current Research And Innovation 73
Potential Improvements In Implant Design 75
Promising Treatments For Hearing Restoration . 76
The Changing Landscape Of Cochlear Implant Technology 78
Conclusion 81
THE END 84

ABOUT THIS BOOK

The "Complete Guide to Understanding Cochlear Implant Surgery" is an essential resource for anybody contemplating or receiving cochlear implant surgery, as well as their families and caregivers. This comprehensive handbook covers all elements of the cochlear implant experience, from pre-operative planning to long-term maintenance and beyond.

Chapter 1 provides an informative introduction to cochlear implant surgery, explaining the complicated workings of this wonderful device. It clarifies the notion of cochlear implants, describing how they work and outlining the eligibility requirements. Furthermore, readers obtain useful insights into the surgical process itself, which alleviates any concerns they may have.

Chapter 2 walks readers through the critical stages needed in preparing for cochlear implant surgery. This part ensures that people go into their surgical journey with information and confidence, from the first consultation and assessment to pre-operative medical testing and mental preparedness.

Chapter 3 delves into the surgical technique itself, providing readers with a full roadmap of what to anticipate throughout the surgery. From anesthetic and incision to implant device placement and post-operative care, every aspect of the operation is thoroughly explained, allowing patients to approach the process with informed consent.

Chapter 4 digs into the essential stages of recovery and rehabilitation, focusing on immediate post-operative care, the healing process, and the activation of the cochlear implant. Furthermore, readers are provided with techniques for auditory training and rehabilitation programs, which will help them move to a world of sound.

Recognizing the value of educated decision-making, Chapter 5 discusses the possible risks and problems of cochlear implant surgery. This section enables users to manage their implant journey with caution and care by identifying surgical risks, device-related problems, and risk-mitigation options.

Chapter 6 walks readers through the process of adapting to life with a cochlear implant. Expectations are contrasted with reality, and readers are given communication skills, speech therapy resources, and lifestyle changes to improve their hearing experience.

Chapter 7 focuses on the maintenance and care of the cochlear implant, providing readers with essential insights into daily care routines, resolving frequent concerns, and the need for regular device checkups. This portion preserves the implant's durability and effectiveness, protecting your investment in auditory improvement.

Chapter 8 focuses on optimizing the advantages of cochlear implantation by highlighting the necessity of ongoing auditory training, experimenting with advanced features, and connecting with support networks. Individuals may achieve new levels of auditory experience and involvement by fully using their implants.

Financial issues and insurance coverage are thoroughly discussed in Chapter 9, providing readers with information on the cost of surgery, insurance coverage alternatives, and accessible financial aid programs. This clause assures that people may get cochlear implantation without incurring unnecessary financial burdens, promoting fair access to auditory rehabilitation.

Finally, Chapter 10 provides a fascinating view into the future of cochlear implant technology by delving into current research, prospective enhancements, and developing treatments for hearing restoration. Readers who remain up to date on the newest developments are better able to make educated choices regarding their auditory health and well-being.

In essence, the "Complete Guide to Understanding Cochlear Implant Surgery" is a beacon of information and empowerment for anyone starting on their cochlear implant journey. From origin to completion, this book is a constant companion, showing the route to aural improvement and enhancing lives via the gift of sound.

CHAPTER 1

Introduction To Cochlear Implant Surgery

What Is A Cochlear Implant?

A cochlear implant is a sophisticated electronic device meant to restore hearing to those who have severe to profound hearing loss and cannot benefit from regular hearing aids. Unlike hearing aids, which enhance sound, cochlear implants bypass damaged areas of the ear and directly stimulate the auditory nerve, enabling users to experience sound.

How Do Cochlear Implants Work?

Understanding how a cochlear implant works requires knowledge of the ear's anatomy as well as the sound transmission mechanism. Sound enters the outer ear, passes down the ear canal, and causes the eardrum to vibrate. These vibrations are subsequently transported to the cochlea, which is a spiral-shaped organ in the inner ear that contains fluid. Thousands of microscopic hair cells in the cochlea transform sound vibrations into electrical impulses that go to the brain via the auditory nerve.

Individuals with severe to profound hearing loss have damaged or non-functional hair cells, which prevent them from converting sound vibrations into electrical impulses. A cochlear implant stimulates the hearing nerve directly with electrical impulses, bypassing the damaged hair cells.

To put it simply, a cochlear implant has two primary components: an exterior piece and an inside portion. The exterior part consists of a microphone, speech processor, and transmitter coil that is worn behind the ear or on the body. The microphone collects up sound, which the speech processor converts into digital signals. The transmitter coil transmits these impulses to the implant's interior components.

The internal part, which is surgically implanted under the skin behind the ear, includes a receiver stimulator and an array of electrodes injected into the cochlea. The receiver-stimulator accepts digital signals from the external processor and turns them into electrical impulses. These impulses are subsequently sent to the electrodes, which activate the auditory nerve fibers inside the cochlea. The brain interprets these electrical impulses as sound, enabling the person to hear even if their hair cells are destroyed or non-functional.

Who Is Suitable For Cochlear Implant Surgery?

Cochlear implant surgery is often suggested for those who have severe to profound sensorineural hearing loss in both ears and do not respond well to hearing aids. Candidates for cochlear implantation are thoroughly evaluated by a team of audiologists, otolaryngologists (ear, nose, and throat experts), and other healthcare professionals to establish their appropriateness for the operation.

The level of hearing loss, the individual's speech recognition ability, their general health and medical history, and their desire and expectations for the result of the operation are all important considerations for assessing eligibility. While cochlear implants may considerably enhance communication and quality of life for many people with hearing loss, they are not appropriate for everyone, and candidacy decisions are made on an individual basis.

Overview Of The Surgical Procedure

Cochlear implant surgery is a generally safe and normal technique that is carried out under general anesthesia. It usually takes two to four hours and is done by a skilled otolaryngologist (ENT surgeon) who specializes in cochlear implantation.

An incision is made behind the ear, and a tiny aperture is produced in the mastoid bone to get access to the cochlea. The surgeon gently inserts the electrode array into the cochlea and places the receiver stimulator under the skin behind the ear. Once the implant is safely in place, the incision is closed and the implant's exterior components are attached.

Following surgery, patients are frequently admitted to the hospital overnight for monitoring before being discharged the following day. Recovery times vary from person to person, but most people may return to regular activities within a few days to a week after surgery.

After the surgical site has healed, an audiologist activates and programs the external components of the cochlear implant during a series of follow-up sessions. This programming procedure includes modifying the speech processor's parameters to enhance sound perception and clarity for each particular user.

CHAPTER 2

Preparing For Cochlear Implant Surgery

The Consultation And Evaluation Process

Before having cochlear implant surgery, people usually meet with an ear, nose, and throat (ENT) doctor or audiologist who specializes in cochlear implants. During the first appointment, the healthcare professional will do a comprehensive exam to establish if the patient is a good candidate for cochlear implantation.

The examination procedure often includes a battery of tests to examine the individual's hearing abilities, including pure tone audiometry, speech audiometry, and perhaps auditory brainstem response (ABR) testing. These tests assist the healthcare professional in determining the level of the patient's hearing loss and if a cochlear implant would be advantageous.

Furthermore, the healthcare professional will examine the patient's medical history, including any past ear operations or medical disorders that might impact the success of the cochlear implant surgery. Patients must submit extensive information about their medical history during this session to ensure a safe and effective surgical result.

Furthermore, the meeting allows patients to ask questions and express any concerns they may have concerning the cochlear implant operation. Patients should feel comfortable sharing their expectations, lifestyle, and aspirations with their healthcare professionals to ensure that cochlear implantation is a good fit for them.

Medical Tests And Assessments

Following the first consultation, patients will go through a battery of medical tests and exams to determine their eligibility for cochlear implant surgery. These tests allow healthcare practitioners to learn more about the patient's general health and any possible dangers related to surgery.

Patients may receive the following medical tests and assessments:

1. **Imaging Studies:** Magnetic resonance imaging (MRI) or computed tomography (CT) scans may be performed to analyze the inner ear structures and see if any anomalies might impede the cochlear implant placement.

2. Blood tests may be performed to examine the patient's general health and to detect any underlying medical issues that might impact the surgical result.

3. **Balance Testing:** Because the inner ear is important for balance, patients may undergo balance testing to examine their vestibular function and determine whether they are at risk of developing balance difficulties following cochlear implant surgery.

4. Psychological examination: In certain situations, individuals may be subjected to a psychological examination to determine their mental health and emotional fitness for cochlear implantation. This examination ensures that patients have reasonable expectations and are prepared to face the obstacles of hearing rehabilitation after surgery.

Preoperative Instructions and Guidelines

Patients will get extensive pre-operative instructions and recommendations to assist them prepare for their cochlear implant operation. These instructions usually include:

1. Medication Guidelines: Patients may be encouraged to discontinue certain drugs, such as blood thinners, in the days before surgery to lessen the risk of bleeding during the operation.

2. Fasting Instructions: Patients are often recommended to fast for some time before surgery to avoid anesthesia-related issues.

3. Hygiene Protocol: To limit the risk of infection, patients may be advised to shower and wash their hair with a specific antibacterial shampoo the night before or morning of operation.

4. Arrangements for Transportation and Accompaniment: Patients are often recommended to plan for transportation to and from the hospital on the day of surgery, since they may be unable to drive themselves home. Furthermore, having a friend or family member accompany them to the hospital might provide emotional support and aid throughout the pre-operative period.

Following these pre-operative recommendations ensures that patients are in the best possible condition for surgery and lowers the chance of problems.

Mental And Emotional Preparation

Undergoing cochlear implant surgery may be a momentous choice for people, eliciting a variety of emotions. Individuals must engage in mental and emotional preparation to deal with the obstacles and uncertainties of the surgery.

Patients may find it beneficial to:

1. **Educate Them:** Learning as much as possible about cochlear implants, the surgical procedure, and what to anticipate after surgery helps reduce anxiety and enable patients to make educated choices regarding their care.

2. **Seek Support:** Connecting with others who have had cochlear implant surgery or joining hearing loss support groups may give helpful emotional and practical guidance.

3. Practice Relaxation Techniques: Deep breathing, meditation, and yoga may all help decrease tension and foster a feeling of calm in the run-up to surgery.

4. Communicate with Healthcare professionals: Open communication with healthcare professionals about worries, concerns, and expectations may help patients feel less anxious and more supported throughout the pre-operative process.

Patients who take proactive actions to improve their mental and emotional well-being may face cochlear implant surgery with confidence and resilience, setting the way for a smoother recovery and successful hearing rehabilitation journey.

CHAPTER 3

Surgical Procedure

Anesthesia And Incision

Before getting into the complexities of cochlear implant surgery, it's critical to grasp the first stages, which begin with anesthesia and the incision. Anesthesia is critical for keeping the patient comfortable and safe during the treatment. Typically, general anesthesia is used, which means the patient is completely asleep and uninformed of the procedure. This guarantees that they are pain-free and fully relaxed.

Once the patient is anesthetized, the surgeon makes an incision behind the ear. This incision is meticulously constructed to allow the best access to the cochlea while minimizing scarring and other issues. The surgeon takes great care to produce a precise incision, generally in the form of a tiny curve or "C," which allows for simple access to the underlying structures while minimizing harm to adjacent tissues.

An incision is made through the epidermis and underlying tissue to expose the mastoid bone. This bone is then gently drilled away to reveal the cochlea, which is deep inside the inner ear. To guarantee the best potential result for the patient, the surgeon must carefully negotiate these fragile structures.

Installation Of The Implant Device

The implant device is then placed once the cochlea has been exposed during the surgical operation. This gadget has two major components: an internal receiver-stimulator and an external speech processor. The internal receiver-stimulator is surgically implanted in the mastoid bone behind the ear, while the external speech processor is worn outside the ear and coupled to the internal device via a magnet.

The surgeon carefully places the internal receiver stimulator into the mastoid bone, ensuring that it is tightly fastened and appropriately aligned with the cochlea. This phase requires accuracy and attention to detail to prevent harming any surrounding structures and guarantee that the implant functions optimally.

Once the internal device is in place, the surgeon attaches it to the electrode array, which is then put into the cochlea. This array comprises several small electrodes that activate the auditory nerve fibers inside the cochlea, enabling the patient to sense sound.

Secure The Electrode Array

Once the implant device is in situ, the surgeon gently inserts the electrode array into the cochlea. This delicate process requires accuracy and experience to guarantee that the electrodes are appropriately positioned and capable of stimulating the auditory nerve fibers adequately.

Once the electrode array is in place, the surgeon fastens it to the surrounding tissue to prevent movement or displacement. Sutures and tissue adhesives are often used to guarantee that the array stays in the proper place inside the cochlea.

Closing The Incision And Postoperative Care

Once the electrode array is firmly in place, the surgeon closes the incision with sutures or surgical staples. This is done with extreme caution to ensure appropriate wound healing and minimal scarring. Once the incision is closed, the patient is sent to a recovery area where they will be carefully followed while they awaken from anesthesia.

Post-operative care is critical for a satisfactory result of cochlear implant surgery. Patients are usually given pain medication to alleviate their agony and antibiotics to avoid infection.

They will also be given information on how to care for the incision site and how to use and maintain their new cochlear implant.

Patients will have follow-up meetings with their surgeon in the days and weeks after surgery to check their progress and alter the implant settings as needed. With adequate care and rehabilitation, most patients see considerable improvements in their hearing and quality of life after cochlear implant surgery.

CHAPTER 4

Recovery And Rehabilitation

Immediate Post-Op Care

Patients are normally brought to a recovery center immediately after cochlear implant surgery, where medical personnel check their vital signs and ensure their comfort. Patients may have soreness, edema, or dizziness after surgery, although these symptoms are usually managed with medicine.

Patients are urged to keep the surgical site clean and dry, and they may be advised to avoid activities that might cause pressure on the head, such as bending or carrying heavy things. It is critical to carefully follow the surgeon's post-operative care recommendations to promote good healing and reduce the chance of problems.

In rare situations, patients may be required to spend the night in the hospital for monitoring, particularly if their recovery is uncertain. Throughout this period, medical personnel will continue to check the patient's status and give any required treatment or assistance.

Healing Process And Follow-Up Appointments

The recovery process after cochlear implant surgery usually encompasses multiple phases. Patients may suffer swelling, bruising, or discomfort around the surgical site for many days or weeks after the treatment. It is critical to keep the region clean and dry to avoid infection and encourage healing.

Follow-up sessions with the surgeon are essential throughout the recovery period. These sessions enable the surgeon to monitor the patient's development, evaluate the implant's health, and handle any issues or difficulties that may emerge. Patients may also be subjected to imaging tests, such as X-rays or MRI scans, to confirm that the implant is adequately working and positioned.

During follow-up sessions, patients may ask any questions or express concerns regarding their recovery or the operation of their cochlear implant. The surgeon and other members of the medical team will give patients support and assistance to ensure a good recovery.

Activation Of The Cochlear Implant

Once the surgical site has healed, patients will go through a procedure known as "activation" to start utilizing their cochlear implant. This usually happens several weeks following surgery, when the edema has reduced and the implant has had time to merge with the surrounding tissue.

During the activation phase, an audiologist or hearing expert will program the implant to ensure that it works properly and produces the best sound quality.

This may include modifying different parameters, such as volume levels and frequency ranges, to meet the patient's specific requirements and preferences.

The activation session is a thrilling milestone for patients because it represents the start of their path to hearing with a cochlear implant. However, it is critical to have reasonable expectations for the early outcomes, since it might take time for the brain to adapt to the new method of hearing and for patients to completely acclimate to utilizing the implant.

Auditory Training And Rehabilitation Programs

Following activation, patients will often go through auditory training and rehabilitation programs to help them acclimate to hearing with a cochlear implant. These programs are intended to help patients learn the skills and tactics necessary to make the most of their new hearing abilities.

Auditory training may include activities that increase speech perception, sound identification, and listening comprehension. Patients may also consult with a speech-language pathologist to create communication skills and increase their ability to comprehend and interact with others.

Counseling and support services may be included in rehabilitation programs to assist patients in dealing with the emotional and psychological elements of hearing loss and cochlear implantation. To gain the greatest results, patients must actively participate in their rehabilitation process and practice daily.

Overall, healing and rehabilitation after cochlear implant surgery need patience, perseverance, and support from both medical experts and family members. With time and effort, many people may significantly improve their hearing and quality of life.

CHAPTER 5

Potential Risks And Complications
Surgery Risks And Precautions

Before entering into the complexity of cochlear implant surgery, it is critical to understand the dangers and precautions involved. Cochlear implantation, like any other operation, has inherent hazards, although technological developments and surgical procedures have dramatically lowered these risks over time.

One of the biggest hazards of cochlear implant surgery is infection. As with any invasive surgery, there is a danger of introducing germs into the body and causing illness. Surgeons make painstaking efforts to reduce this risk, such as thoroughly sterilizing equipment and operating rooms and providing antibiotics before, during, and after operation.

Another possible danger is injury to neighboring tissues inside the ear, such as the facial nerve or the balancing structures. Surgeons must negotiate sensitive anatomy throughout the treatment, and although inadvertent harm is uncommon, it does occur. To reduce this danger, surgeons get significant training and use modern imaging methods to accurately find and avoid these structures.

Another issue with cochlear implant surgery is hemorrhage or excessive bleeding. While bleeding is usually little, some medical conditions or drugs might heighten the risk. To reduce this risk, surgeons may take extra measures, such as stopping blood thinners before surgery.

Device-Related Complications

Once the implant is in place, there may be issues with the device itself. One typical concern is device failure or malfunction, which may be caused by technical faults or implant damage. While current cochlear implants are quite dependable, failures may occur, needing device replacement or repair.

Another device-related issue is device extrusion or migration, in which the implant moves away from its intended place inside the cochlea. This might arise as a result of poor fixation or trauma to the implant site. Surgeons take steps during the first installation to reduce the danger of extrusion, although it may occur on rare occasions.

Strategies For Minimizing Risk

To reduce the risks of cochlear implant surgery, doctors use a range of tactics before, during, and after the process. Preoperative assessments assist surgeons detect any underlying medical issues that may raise the risk of complications, enabling them to take the necessary safeguards.

During surgery, great attention to detail and perfect surgical technique are critical for reducing risks. Surgeons use modern imaging equipment, such as CT scans and MRI, to map the ear's architecture and arrange the surgical procedure.

Intraoperative monitoring tools, such as facial nerve monitoring, contribute to the safety of adjacent tissues throughout the treatment.

Postoperative care is equally critical in reducing risks and consequences. Patients are continuously examined following surgery for symptoms of infection or bleeding. Antibiotics may be recommended to prevent infection, and patients are taught adequate wound care practices to reduce the likelihood of problems.

Long-Term Monitoring And Management

Even after successful implementation, long-term monitoring and management are critical for improving results and reducing risks. Regular follow-up meetings with an audiologist and an otolaryngologist are required to check device operation and resolve any problems that may occur.

Routine maintenance of external components, such as the speech processor and microphone, helps to guarantee the device's best operation. Patients are taught troubleshooting procedures and urged to rapidly report any changes in hearing or device operation.

Furthermore, continued rehabilitation and auditory training are critical for reaping the full advantages of cochlear implantation. Patients work closely with speech-language pathologists to improve their auditory abilities and adjust to hearing with the implant. Regular contact with the healthcare team allows for necessary revisions to the implant's programming.

By following these long-term monitoring and management measures, patients may enhance their hearing and quality of life while reducing the risks and difficulties associated with cochlear implant surgery.

CHAPTER 6

Adjusting To Life With A Cochlear Implant

Expectations Vs Reality

When contemplating cochlear implant surgery, it is critical to understand the expectations against the reality of the procedure and results. While many people expect rapid, significant hearing gains, the reality is generally more complicated. Cochlear implants may alter people's lives, but the path to optimum hearing is gradual.

One widespread assumption is that hearing with a cochlear implant will be equal to normal hearing. However, it is critical to understand that cochlear implants provide a unique audio experience. Initially, sounds may seem distorted or strange as your brain adapts to interpreting implant information. Understanding this might help you manage expectations and avoid frustration throughout the adoption phase.

Anticipation is that cochlear implants would provide flawless hearing. While they may greatly increase hearing skills, they may not fully simulate natural hearing, especially in busy areas or with specific kinds of noises. Managing expectations entails acknowledging the limits of cochlear implants while enjoying the tremendous gains they provide in everyday life.

Adapting To Sound Perception

Getting used to sound perception with a cochlear implant is a long process that takes patience and persistence. Initially, sounds may be overpowering or confused while your brain learns to process implant information. Allow yourself time to adjust to these new feelings and practice listening in various settings.

Gradual exposure to varied sounds and situations is one approach to learning to perceive sound. Begin with tranquil, familiar environments and gradually progress to increasingly complex aural stimuli. This stepwise method helps your brain to gradually acclimate to hearing sounds from the implant.

Auditory training activities, which are performed by audiologists or speech therapists, are also beneficial. These activities are meant to help you interpret speech and distinguish distinct sounds. Consistent practice may considerably improve your capacity to receive and comprehend auditory information with your cochlear implant.

Communication Strategies And Speech Therapy

Effective communication methods are required to maximize the advantages of cochlear implants. Speech therapy is essential for establishing these skills and enhancing speech comprehension and output.

Speech therapists work with people to enhance their listening abilities, speech clarity, and language development.

Visual clues, such as lip-reading and facial expressions, are typical communication approaches that may help people interpret speech. Learning to depend on visual signals in combination with auditory information may improve communication efficacy, especially in difficult listening situations.

Another effective method is to advocate for yourself and educate people about your cochlear implant. Informing friends, family, and colleagues about your communication requirements and preferences may lead to easier interactions and more understanding and support.

Lifestyle Changes And Support Networks

Adjusting to life with a cochlear implant sometimes entails making lifestyle changes to fit your hearing requirements.

This might involve employing assistive listening equipment, such as FM systems or captioned phones, to aid communication in a variety of situations. Furthermore, forming a support network of friends, family, and other cochlear implant patients may give vital emotional and practical help.

Joining support groups or online forums for cochlear implant recipients helps you to connect with people who share your experiences and problems. These communities may provide helpful insights, support, and information for living with a cochlear implant.

To summarize, adjusting to life with a cochlear implant entails controlling expectations, adapting to sound perception, creating effective communication skills via speech therapy, and making lifestyle changes while establishing a strong support system. Individuals who understand and embrace these parts of the cochlear implant experience may optimize their hearing capacity and improve their overall quality of life.

CHAPTER 7

Maintenance And Care For The Cochlear Implant

Daily Care Routine For External Components

Maintaining the exterior components of your cochlear implant is critical to maintaining its life and good function. A regular care practice helps to avoid damage and maintain cleanliness. Here's a quick instruction to care for the exterior components.

1. Cleaning: Begin by carefully cleaning the cochlear implant's exterior pieces with a soft, dry cloth. Avoid using liquid cleansers or abrasive agents, since they might harm the sensitive components. Pay extra attention to places where perspiration or grime might gather.

2. **Battery Management:** Regularly check the battery state to ensure that it is fully charged. Depending on the kind of cochlear implant you have, the battery may need to be recharged regularly or replaced with disposable batteries. Always have extra batteries with you, particularly while traveling.

3. Moisture may destroy the cochlear implant's electrical components. Use a protective cover or sleeve while swimming or bathing. Also, try using a dehumidifier to remove moisture from the device overnight.

4. **Securing the Processor:** Make sure the processor is properly fastened to your clothes or worn comfortably behind your ear. To hold it in place during everyday activities, use the manufacturer-provided clips or accessories.

5. **Check for Damage:** Inspect the exterior components regularly for indications of damage or wear. If you

find any cracks, scratches, or loose pieces, call your audiologist or cochlear implant expert for help.

By adding these basic procedures into your everyday routine, you may efficiently maintain your cochlear implant's exterior components and increase its longevity.

Troubleshooting: Common Issues

Despite good care and maintenance, you may sometimes have problems with your cochlear implant. Knowing how to troubleshoot common issues might help you resolve them more quickly and efficiently. Below are some frequent difficulties and troubleshooting steps:

1. No Sound: If you aren't hearing anything from your cochlear implant, check the battery to make sure it's fully charged or replace it. If the battery is not the problem, examine the connections between the external components and the implant site to verify

they are secure. If the issue continues, call your audiologist for more help.

2. Feedback or whistling sounds might occur if the microphone or receiver coil is not properly positioned. Adjust the positioning of the exterior components to reduce interference and guarantee a good fit. Avoid covering the microphone or receiver coil with clothes or hair, since this might result in feedback.

3. **Discomfort or Irritation:** If you feel discomfort or irritation at the implant site or behind your ear, look for pressure points or skin irritation. Adjust the processor's position or use cushioning cushions to relieve pressure and increase comfort.

4. **Loss of Connection:** External components may lose contact with the implant site owing to mobility or environmental variables. Check the connections and make sure that all wires are properly plugged in. Avoid rapid movements or heavy perspiration, which might interrupt the connection.

5. Inconsistent Performance: If you observe inconsistent performance or changes in sound quality, conduct a system reset by shutting off the processor and then restarting it after a few seconds. If the issue continues, speak with your audiologist for further troubleshooting and adjustments.

By following these troubleshooting methods, you may efficiently handle frequent difficulties with your cochlear implant and ensure its continued usage.

Battery Management And Replacement

Proper battery management is critical for maintaining continuous usage of your cochlear implant. Depending on the kind of implant, you may use rechargeable or disposable batteries. Here's how to properly monitor and replace your cochlear implant batteries:

1. Rechargeable Batteries: If your cochlear implant requires rechargeable batteries, make sure they are completely charged before usage. Follow the manufacturer's charging guidelines and prevent overcharging the batteries, which might shorten their lifetime. Bring a portable charger with you for convenience, particularly while traveling.

2. Disposable Batteries: If your cochlear implant requires disposable batteries, maintain a supply of new batteries on hand at all times. To avoid disruptions in sound processing, check the battery state regularly and replace it as necessary. Dispose of old batteries correctly by local rules.

3. Battery Life: Check the battery life indicator on your processor to see when it's time to recharge or replace the batteries. Rechargeable batteries normally last a full day before having to be recharged, however, throwaway batteries may last several days to a week, depending on use.

4. Emergency Preparedness: Always have extra batteries with you, particularly while traveling or in an emergency. To ensure their efficacy, keep them cool and dry, away from direct sunshine and harsh temperatures.

5. Battery Replacement: To replace the batteries in your cochlear implant, follow the manufacturer's instructions. When handling batteries, use care to prevent damage or injury. If you have any problems or have concerns concerning battery replacement, contact your audiologist or cochlear implant expert for help.

By correctly monitoring and changing your cochlear implant batteries, you can ensure your device's continuing usage and excellent performance.

Regular Device Checks And Maintenance

Regular check-ups and maintenance are required to ensure the long-term operation and effectiveness of your cochlear implant. Here's why they're crucial and what you should anticipate from these appointments:

1. **Monitoring Performance:** At frequent check-ups, your audiologist will evaluate the performance of your cochlear implant device and make any required changes to improve sound quality and clarity. They may administer a variety of exams, including speech perception tests and device programming changes.

2. **Troubleshooting Issues:** If you have any difficulties or concerns with your cochlear implant, frequent check-ups allow you to address them quickly. Your audiologist can diagnose typical problems, such as feedback or uneven performance, and make any required changes or repairs.

3. **Device Maintenance:** Your audiologist will also do regular maintenance on your cochlear implant system to ensure that all components work properly. This may involve cleaning and examining the exterior components, ensuring the implant site's integrity, and replacing old or broken elements.

4. Counseling and assistance: Regular check-ups provide the chance for counseling and assistance. Your audiologist can advise you on how to properly use and care for your cochlear implant, as well as answer any questions or concerns you may have regarding your hearing rehabilitation journey.

5. Long-term Monitoring: As you use your cochlear implant, frequent check-ups enable your audiologist to monitor your development and make any required changes to guarantee your continuing success. They may also provide advice on long-term hearing restoration objectives and tactics.

You can get the most out of your cochlear implant by going to frequent check-ups and following your audiologist's maintenance and care instructions.

CHAPTER 8

Maximizing The Benefits Of Cochlear Implants

Continued Auditory Training And Rehabilitation

After cochlear implant surgery, the path to greater hearing does not stop there. In reality, it's just the beginning. Continued auditory training and rehabilitation are critical for optimizing the advantages of cochlear implants.

Imagine your brain as a garden, with your new cochlear implant serving as the seeds. To guarantee that those seeds develop into healthy plants, you must care for them regularly. Auditory training is like watering and nourishing those seedlings. It consists of workouts and activities meant to help your brain adjust to the new method of processing sound.

Rehabilitation is the sunshine that enables those seeds to flourish. It involves sessions with speech therapists and audiologists who will walk you through activities to enhance your listening, speech comprehension, and general communication skills. These sessions are targeted to your unique requirements and development, ensuring that you gradually improve your hearing.

Exploring Advanced Features And Accessories

Cochlear implants provide several sophisticated features and accessories that may help you hear even better. From Bluetooth connection to specialist microphones, these gadgets expand the options for cochlear implant users.

One such function is the ability to link your cochlear implant to other devices wirelessly via Bluetooth. This enables you to stream audio straight to your implant from your smartphone, television, or computer, resulting in better and more immersive sound.

Another handy item is a remote microphone. This little gadget may be worn by a conversation partner or positioned in a strategic spot to take up sound more efficiently in difficult listening circumstances, such as loud restaurants or packed classrooms.

Exploring these sophisticated features and accessories may greatly increase your capacity to communicate and interact with the world around you, making daily tasks more pleasurable and doable.

Strategies For Challenged Listening Environments

Navigating difficult hearing conditions may be difficult for anybody, but particularly for those who have cochlear implants. However, with the appropriate techniques in place, you can overcome these challenges and prosper in any environment.

One useful method is to use visual clues wherever feasible. This might include observing the speaker's lips or facial expressions to enhance the aural information you're getting. Visual signals may give useful information and fill in any gaps in your hearing.

Another effective strategy is to advocate for yourself and your demands. Don't be hesitant to speak out and express your needs, whether it's asking for concessions in loud environments or suggesting that speakers use clear and precise language.

Furthermore, using active listening strategies, such as summarizing what you've heard or seeking clarification when necessary, may increase comprehension and prevent misconceptions in difficult situations.

By using these tactics and being proactive in regulating your hearing, you will be able to comfortably handle any listening circumstance that arises.

Advocacy And Community Involvement

Being an advocate for oneself and the cochlear implant community as a whole is critical for raising awareness, increasing access to resources, and cultivating a supportive community.

One method to advocate for yourself is to remain up to date on developments in cochlear implant technology and research. By educating yourself, you may make more informed choices regarding your care and participate in conversations about the future of cochlear implants.

Community engagement is another critical component of advocacy. Joining support groups, attending cochlear implant events, and sharing your own experiences may all give essential support and encouragement to those going through a similar path.

Advocating for regulatory reforms and more financing for cochlear implant programs may also assist in guaranteeing that this life-changing technology is available to everyone who needs it.

By actively participating in advocacy and community participation, you may help define the future of cochlear implantation and improve the lives of people with hearing loss.

CHAPTER 9

Financial Considerations And Insurance Coverage

Cost Of Cochlear Implant Surgery

The cost of cochlear implant surgery varies based on various variables, including the hospital or clinic where the operation is conducted, the surgeon's fees, the kind of implant device utilized, and any extra services or tests necessary before or after surgery. On average, cochlear implant surgery costs between $30,000 and $50,000 for each ear. This cost generally covers the surgical surgery, the implant device, initial programming and activation, and follow-up sessions.

Individuals contemplating cochlear implant surgery should understand the breakdown of these prices and ask about any extra charges that may occur. Some hospitals or clinics may provide financing alternatives or payment plans to assist patients in managing the financial burden of surgery.

Insurance Coverage And Reimbursement

Many health insurance policies, including Medicare and Medicaid, pay for part or all of the cost of cochlear implant surgery. However, coverage policies vary greatly across insurance companies and individual plans. Some insurance plans may pay for the full operation and accompanying expenditures, while others may require the patient to pay a part of the cost out of cash.

Before having cochlear implant surgery, patients should contact their insurance carrier to assess their coverage and any out-of-pocket expenditures they may incur. Insurance companies may need prior permission or paperwork from a healthcare practitioner before approving coverage for surgery.

Financial Assistance Programs

Individuals who do not have appropriate insurance coverage or cannot pay the out-of-pocket fees involved with cochlear implant surgery might benefit from financial assistance programs. These programs may be provided by government agencies, non-profit groups, or cochlear implant device manufacturers.

One such initiative is the Aid for Hearing Loss program, which offers financial aid to those with hearing loss who need cochlear implant surgery but cannot pay the price. Furthermore, some manufacturers provide financial aid or patient assistance programs to help people pay for their implant devices or associated fees.

Planning For Long-Term Maintenance Expenses

In addition to the initial costs of cochlear implant surgery, people should think about the long-term maintenance fees that come with having a cochlear implant. These expenditures may include continuous medical treatment, such as frequent check-ups with an audiologist or otolaryngologist, as well as the cost of replacement implant components or accessories.

Some insurance plans may cover regular maintenance and replacement components for cochlear implants, while others may require patients to pay for these costs themselves. Individuals seeking cochlear implant surgery must include these long-term maintenance fees in their financial planning.

Individuals can make informed decisions about pursuing cochlear implant surgery as a treatment option for hearing loss by understanding the costs associated with the procedure, navigating insurance coverage and reimbursement policies, researching financial assistance programs, and planning for long-term maintenance expenses.

CHAPTER 10

Future Developments And Emerging Technology

Current Research And Innovation

Cochlear implant surgery is a continually growing discipline, with new research and novel improvements. Researchers and medical experts are always looking for new approaches and technologies to enhance the efficacy and results of cochlear implants.

One aspect of the ongoing study is focused on improving the surgical technique itself. Surgeons are looking at less invasive procedures to decrease surgical trauma and enhance patient recovery periods. This includes developments in surgical equipment and techniques that enable more accurate placement of implant electrodes inside the cochlea.

Another area of ongoing research is the creation of improved implant technologies. Engineers and scientists are working on developing implants that are smaller, more durable, and more effective in stimulating the auditory nerve. This may include the use of innovative materials or electronics to improve the implant's function and lifetime.

Furthermore, researchers are looking at novel methods for enhancing the programming and customization of cochlear implants. This entails creating algorithms and software that can change stimulation settings to each patient's specific demands and preferences. Clinicians may increase speech perception and auditory performance by fine-tuning the implant's settings.

Overall, current research in cochlear implant surgery focuses on improving surgical technique, upgrading implant technology, and fine-tuning implant programming and personalization to maximize results for individuals with hearing loss.

Potential Improvements In Implant Design

In the drive to improve cochlear implant technology, researchers are looking at several ways to improve the architecture of the implants themselves. These possible advancements seek to make cochlear implants smaller, more efficient, and more biocompatible, resulting in improved results for patients.

One area of research is the creation of thinner, more flexible electrode arrays. Traditional cochlear implants include electrode arrays that are placed into the cochlea to stimulate the auditory nerve. Researchers expect that developing these arrays smaller and more flexible would enhance the surgical insertion procedure and reduce stress on the delicate components of the inner ear.

Another area of study is the use of new materials to manufacture electrodes. Engineers are looking at materials that are more biocompatible and can offer electrical stimulation to the auditory nerve. By improving the materials used in cochlear implants, researchers hope to increase the devices' long-term durability and function.

Additionally, researchers are looking at methods to enhance the energy efficiency of cochlear implants. This involves looking into novel power sources, like as rechargeable batteries or energy harvesting technologies, to extend the implant's lifetime and eliminate the need for frequent battery replacements.

Overall, future advancements in implant design offer the possibility of making cochlear implants smaller, more efficient, and more dependable, resulting in improved results for people with hearing loss.

Promising Treatments For Hearing Restoration

In addition to cochlear implants, researchers are looking at a variety of potential hearing restoration techniques.

These treatments attempt to cure various forms of hearing loss and may provide alternative treatment choices for those who are not suitable for cochlear implantation.

One field of study is gene therapy for hearing loss. Scientists are looking for methods to transfer therapeutic genes to the inner ear to repair or replace damaged hair cells or auditory nerve fibers. This method has the potential to restore hearing in those who have certain inherited kinds of hearing loss or who have acquired hearing loss owing to injury to the inner ear.

Stem cell treatment is another potential approach to hearing repair. Researchers are investigating the ability of stem cells to repair or replace damaged hair cells and auditory nerve cells in the inner ear. Scientists want to create novel hearing loss therapies that restore auditory function in people with sensorineural hearing loss by using stem cells' regeneration ability.

Furthermore, researchers are looking at the use of auditory brainstem implants (ABIs) for hearing restoration in those with auditory nerve loss. ABIs, unlike cochlear implants, activate auditory circuits in the brainstem rather than the cochlea. This method may provide a solution for those who have severe to profound sensorineural hearing loss and are not candidates for cochlear implantation.

Overall, potential hearing restoration methods provide hope to those who have hearing loss but may not benefit from typical cochlear implants. Researchers want to discover new therapies for hearing loss by investigating newer procedures such as gene therapy, stem cells, and auditory brainstem implants.

The Changing Landscape Of Cochlear Implant Technology

The landscape of cochlear implant technology is continuously changing, as new developments and innovations reshape the industry.

These advancements affect many elements of cochlear implantation, including surgical methods, implant design, and rehabilitation tactics, and have the potential to greatly improve the lives of people with hearing loss.

One prominent tendency in the developing landscape of cochlear implant technology is a move toward individualized and customizable solutions. Clinicians are progressively personalizing cochlear implant programming to each patient's unique requirements and preferences, using modern algorithms and software to improve results. This individualized method allows for more flexibility and fine-tuning of the implant settings, resulting in better speech perception and overall auditory performance.

Another significant advancement is the incorporation of cochlear implants with various assistive devices and technology. Cochlear implant systems are currently being built to easily integrate with smartphones, tablets, and other wireless devices, enabling users to stream audio straight to their implants. This integration improves the accessibility and usefulness of cochlear implants in daily life, allowing users to engage more completely in social, educational, and professional settings.

Furthermore, advances in surgical procedures and implant design are being made in the area of cochlear implantation to improve results and expand the candidate pool. Minimally invasive surgical methods, along with thinner and more flexible electrode arrays, are making cochlear implantation safer and more accessible to a larger variety of patients, including those with challenging anatomical requirements.

Overall, the changing landscape of cochlear implant technology is marked by an emphasis on customization, integration, and innovation. Researchers and clinicians advance the science of cochlear implantation and improve outcomes for people with hearing loss by using modern technology and multidisciplinary cooperation.

Conclusion

Finally, learning about cochlear implant surgery reveals a deep respect for the complex convergence of technology, medicine, and human perseverance. This revolutionary surgery serves as a light of hope for those with profound hearing loss, providing them with a means to reconnect with the world of sound.

At its essence, cochlear implant surgery is a triumph of human creativity and teamwork. From the pioneering efforts of academics and engineers to the skillful hands of surgeons, each stage in the development and deployment of this technology shows a shared dedication to improving the lives of individuals suffering from hearing loss.

A thorough examination of the surgical procedure, from preoperative assessments to postoperative rehabilitation, reveals that success in cochlear implantation is dependent not just on technical skill, but also on customized care and support. The comprehensive approach used by multidisciplinary teams emphasizes the necessity of meeting patients' different demands and problems throughout their journey.

Furthermore, the substantial effects of cochlear implants go well beyond auditory perception. These technologies enable people to achieve their goals and participate more actively in society by recovering their ability to communicate effectively and fully engage in social interactions. increased hearing has a wide-ranging impact on one's life, from increased educational and economic possibilities to expanded relationships and a stronger feeling of belonging.

However, the path to cochlear implantation is not without challenges and uncertainty. From the initial decision-making process to the continuing care of device-related difficulties, patients and their families face many considerations and obstacles. However, it is exactly at these times of uncertainty that the value of comprehensive education and assistance becomes most obvious. By building a collaborative collaboration among patients, caregivers, and healthcare professionals, it is feasible to handle the complications of cochlear implantation with confidence and perseverance.

In the ever-changing environment of medical innovation, cochlear implant surgery is a tribute to the extraordinary advances made in the area of auditory rehabilitation. As technology advances and our knowledge of hearing loss grows, the potential of cochlear implants becomes ever more compelling. By adopting a culture of creativity and sensitivity, we can guarantee that people with hearing impairments not only have the chance to hear but also flourish in a world full of sound and possibilities.

THE END

www.ingramcontent.com/pod-product-compliance
Lightning Source LLC
Chambersburg PA
CBHW071839210526
45479CB00001B/208